ANTI INFLAMMATORY SMOOTHIE

A 1000-Day Diet Cookbook of Healthy Smoothie Recipes for Beginners.

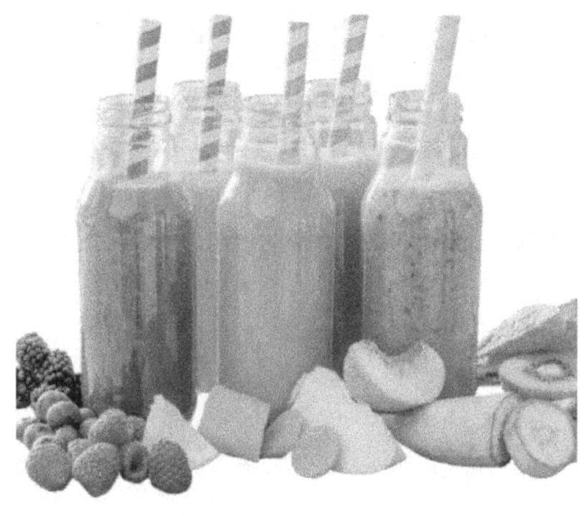

AVELINE WINTER

TABLE OF CONTENT

INTRODUCTION 7

HOW TO USE YOUR ANTI-INFLAMMATORY SMOOTHIE COOKBOOK 9

CHAPTER 1: BERRY BLISS 11

1. Blueberry Burst 11

2. Strawberry Serenity 13

3. Raspberry Radiance 15

4. Mango Mint Magic 17

5. Blackberry Breeze 19

CHAPTER 2: GREEN ELIXIR 21

6. Kale Kiwi Kick 21

7. Spinach Spirulina Splash 23

8. Avocado Alchemy 25

9. Parsley Pineapple Potion 27

10. Cilantro Citrus Crush 29

CHAPTER 3: TROPICAL TRANQUILITY 31

11. Papaya Paradise 31

12. Passionfruit Pleasure 33

13. Guava Glow 35

14. Dragon Fruit Dream 37

15. Coconut Lime Oasis 39

CHAPTER 4: SPICE SYMPHONY 41

16. Turmeric Tonic 41

17. Cinnamon Citrus Sip 43

18. Cardamom Carrot Crush 45

19. Cayenne Mango Mojo 47

20. Rosemary Berry Blast.............................. 49

CHAPTER 5: CITRUS SYMPHONY 51

21. Lemon Lavender Lift................................. 51

22. Orange Ginger Zest................................. 53

23. Grapefruit Green Goddess 55

24. Citrus Basil Bliss.................................... 57

25. Tangerine Turmeric Twist......................... 59

CHAPTER 6: NUTTY NIRVANA 61

26. Almond Joy Delight 61

27. Walnut Wonder 63

28. Cashew Cherry Charm............................. 65

29. Pecan Pumpkin Pleasure 67

30. Hazelnut Hibiscus Hug 69

CHAPTER 7: HERBAL INFUSION............................ 71

31. Peppermint Pineapple Paradise 71

32. Chamomile Citrus Soothe......................... 73

33. Lemongrass Lime Lullaby.......................... 75

34. Basil Berry Breeze.................................. 77

35. Rosehip Raspberry Relaxation 79

CHAPTER 8: FLORAL FUSION 81

36. Hibiscus Honey Harmony 81

37. Lavender Lemonade Lift 83

38. Rose Petal Radiance 85

39. Chamomile Vanilla Velvet 87

40. Jasmine Ginger Jazz 89

CONCLUSION 91

Thrive On, Wellness Seekers 91

I AM READY TO ACCEPT COMFORT AND EASE INTO MY LIFE BY BLENDING HEALTHY FOR A MORE HEALTHIER, HAPPIER AND VIBRANT ME!

INTRODUCTION

Have you ever wondered if a sip could be the remedy to the discomfort that seems to linger with every bite? In a world where inflammation can cast a shadow over our well-being, Aveline Winter invites you on a journey to discover the healing power of her carefully crafted anti-inflammatory smoothies.

Ever felt the subtle yet persistent discomfort that inflammation can bring? Aveline Winter understands. As the creator of this book, she knows the impact it can have on our daily lives. But what if a simple, delicious solution was within reach?

In "Anti-Inflammatory Smoothie by Aveline Winter," she takes you on a vibrant exploration of flavors designed not just to tantalize your taste buds but to soothe the discomfort that inflammation can bring. Aveline has meticulously curated these recipes, drawing from her own experiences and the desire to offer a holistic approach to wellness.

Each recipe within these pages is a testament to Aveline's dedication. Understand the details – every ingredient is listed with precision, every step carefully explained. But it doesn't end there. Discover the nutritional information for every concoction, empowering you to make informed choices for your health.

Aveline understands that one size doesn't fit all. That's why each recipe comes with ingredient substitutes, ensuring that dietary restrictions or allergies don't stand between you and a refreshing, healthful experience. And yes, all these delightful concoctions are tailored for one serving – no fuss, no guesswork.

So, why should you keep on reading this book? Because within these pages lies not just a collection of recipes but a gateway to a more vibrant, healthier life. The benefits extend beyond the delicious sips – they reach into the core of your well-being. Imagine missing out on the chance to alleviate discomfort, boost your energy, and savor the joy of nourishing your body.

As you embark on this journey with Aveline, remember, these aren't just recipes; they are a commitment to your well-being. What you hold in your hands is more than a cookbook – it's an invitation to transform the way you approach your health. Don't let this opportunity pass you by; the first sip into wellness awaits you. Let's sip to a healthier, happier you!

HOW TO USE YOUR ANTI-INFLAMMATORY SMOOTHIE COOKBOOK

Step 1: Explore the Recipes

- Open the cookbook and browse through the various anti-inflammatory smoothie recipes. For each recipe:
- Check out the Detailed Ingredients list to ensure you have everything.
- Follow the Step-by-Step Instructions for a seamless preparation process.

Step 2: Understand the Nutrition

- Learn the nutritional details of each recipe:
- Examine the breakdown of Calories, Proteins, Fats, and Carbs.
- Take note of Fiber and Sugar Content for a health-conscious choice.

Step 3: Customize to Your Taste

- Personalize your smoothie experience:
- Experiment with Ingredient Substitutes suggested for flexibility.
- If you have dietary restrictions or allergies, find Allergy-Friendly Options listed for each smoothie recipe.

Step 4: Perfectly Portioned

- No need for complicated math – all recipes are crafted for a single serving. Just blend and enjoy!

Step 5: Blend, Sip, and Enjoy

- Embrace the joy of blending! Grab your ingredients, follow the instructions, and revel in a refreshing, healthful sip.

Step 6: Keep it Handy

- Bookmark your favorites or snap a quick photo for easy access. Make this cookbook your kitchen companion.

Congratulations! You're now ready to embark on a delightful journey to better health, one smoothie at a time. Happy blending!

CHAPTER 1: BERRY BLISS

1. Blueberry Burst

Ingredients:
- 1 cup fresh or frozen blueberries
- 1 cup fresh spinach leaves
- 1 ½ cups almond milk
- 1 tablespoon chia seeds

Instructions:
1. Wash the blueberries and spinach thoroughly.
2. In a blender, combine the blueberries, spinach, almond milk, and chia seeds.
3. Blend on high speed until the mixture is smooth and well combined.
4. If the smoothie is too thick, add more almond milk in small increments until you reach your desired consistency.
5. Pour the smoothie into a glass and serve.

Nutritional Information:
- Calories: Approximately 200 kcal
- Protein: 7g
- Fat: 10g
- Carbohydrates: 25g
- Fiber: 10g
- Sugar: 10g

Ingredient Substitutes:
- Blueberries: Substitute with raspberries, strawberries, or blackberries.
- Spinach: Swap with kale, Swiss chard, or collard greens.
- Almond Milk: Use coconut milk, soy milk, or oat milk for a different flavor.
- Chia Seeds: Replace with flaxseeds or hemp seeds for an omega-3 boost.

Dietary Needs and Allergies:
- Nut Allergy: Replace almond milk with oat milk or coconut milk.
- Seed Allergy: Omit chia seeds or substitute with ground flaxseeds.
- Low-Carb: Reduce blueberries and replace them with more spinach or kale.
- Diabetic-Friendly: Choose unsweetened almond milk and limit the fruit quantity.
- Lactose Intolerance: Stick with non-dairy milk alternatives.
- Allergic to Berries: Use sliced apples, peaches, or mango as a fruit alternative.

2. Strawberry Serenity

Ingredients:

- 1 cup fresh strawberries, hulled
- 1 cup kale, stems removed
- 1 ½ cups coconut water
- 1 tablespoon flax seeds

Instructions:

1. Wash the strawberries and kale thoroughly.
2. In a blender, combine the strawberries, kale, coconut water, and flaxseeds.
3. Blend on high speed until the mixture is smooth and well combined.
4. If the smoothie is too thick, add more coconut water in small increments until it reaches your taste.
5. Pour the smoothie into a glass and serve.

Nutritional Information:

- Calories: Approximately 150 kcal
- Protein: 5g
- Fat: 5g
- Carbohydrates: 30g
- Fiber: 8g
- Sugar: 15g

Ingredient Substitutes:

- Strawberries: Swap with raspberries, blackberries, or blueberries.
- Kale: Replace with spinach, Swiss chard, or collard greens.

- Coconut Water: Use almond milk, soy milk, or regular water for a lighter taste.
- Flaxseeds: Substitute with chia seeds or hemp seeds for a different omega-3 source.

Dietary Needs and Allergies:
- Nut Allergy: Use water or coconut milk instead of almond milk.
- Seed Allergy: Omit flaxseeds or replace them with sunflower seeds.
- Low-Carb: Reduce strawberries and replace them with more kale or spinach.
- Diabetic-Friendly: Choose unsweetened coconut water and limit the fruit quantity.
- Lactose Intolerance: Opt for non-dairy milk alternatives.
- Allergic to Berries: Use sliced peaches, pineapple, or mango as a fruit alternative.

3. Raspberry Radiance

Ingredients:

- 1 cup fresh raspberries
- 1 cup Swiss chard, stems removed
- ½ cup Greek yogurt
- ½ teaspoon turmeric

Instructions:

1. Wash the raspberries and Swiss chard thoroughly.
2. In a blender, combine the raspberries, Swiss chard, Greek yogurt, and turmeric.
3. Blend on high speed until the mixture is smooth and well combined.
4. Adjust the consistency by adding more Greek yogurt or a splash of water if needed.
5. Pour the smoothie into a glass and serve.

Nutritional Information:

- Calories: Approximately 180 kcal
- Protein: 10g
- Fat: 5g
- Carbohydrates: 25g
- Fiber: 12g
- Sugar: 10g

Ingredient Substitutes:

- Raspberries: Substitute with blackberries, blueberries, or strawberries.
- Swiss Chard: Replace with kale, spinach, or collard greens.

- Greek Yogurt: Use coconut milk yogurt for a dairy-free alternative.
- Turmeric: Swap with ginger for a different anti-inflammatory spice.

Dietary Needs and Allergies:
- Nut Allergy: Use a non-dairy yogurt alternative.
- Lactose Intolerance: Choose lactose-free yogurt or non-dairy yogurt.
- Low-Carb: Reduce the amount of berries and replace them with more leafy greens.
- Diabetic-Friendly: Opt for plain, unsweetened yogurt and limit the fruit quantity.
- Allergic to Berries: Use sliced apples, peaches, or pineapple as a fruit alternative.

4. Mango Mint Magic

Ingredients:

- 1 cup of fresh peeled and diced mango
- 1 handful mint leaves
- ½ cup cucumber, peeled and sliced
- 1 ½ cups coconut milk

Instructions:

1. Wash and peel the mango and cucumber.
2. In a blender, combine the mango, mint leaves, cucumber, and coconut milk.
3. Blend on high speed until the mixture is smooth and well combined.
4. Adjust the thickness by adding more coconut milk if needed.
5. Pour the smoothie into a glass and serve.

Nutritional Information:

- Calories: Approximately 220 kcal
- Protein: 3g
- Fat: 10g
- Carbohydrates: 30g
- Fiber: 6g
- Sugar: 20g

Ingredient Substitutes:
- Mango: Substitute with pineapple, peaches, or apricots.
- Mint Leaves: Replace with basil or cilantro for a different flavor.
- Cucumber: Use zucchini for a milder taste or omit for a sweeter smoothie.
- Coconut Milk: Swap with almond milk, soy milk, or regular water.

Dietary Needs and Allergies:
- Nut Allergy: Choose a non-dairy milk alternative.
- Lactose Intolerance: Opt for lactose-free yogurt or non-dairy yogurt.
- Low-Carb: Reduce the amount of mango and use a lower-carb milk alternative.
- Diabetic-Friendly: Choose unsweetened coconut milk and limit the fruit quantity.
- Allergic to Tropical Fruits: Use berries or stone fruits as a mango alternative.

5. Blackberry Breeze

Ingredients:

- 1 cup fresh blackberries
- ½ cup beetroot, peeled and diced
- 1 cup pineapple, diced
- 1 teaspoon fresh ginger, grated

Instructions:

1. Wash the blackberries and beetroot thoroughly.
2. Peel and dice the beetroot.
3. In a blender, combine the blackberries, beetroot, pineapple, and grated ginger.
4. Blend on high speed until the mixture is smooth and well combined.
5. Adjust the thickness by adding water or a liquid of your choice if needed.
6. Pour the smoothie into a glass and serve.

Nutritional Information:

- Calories: Approximately 160 kcal
- Protein: 3g
- Fat: 1g
- Carbohydrates: 40g
- Fiber: 10g
- Sugar: 25g

Ingredient Substitutes:
- Blackberries: Swap with raspberries, blueberries, or strawberries.
- Beetroot: Replace with carrots or red bell peppers for a different color and taste.
- Pineapple: Use mango, peaches, or oranges for a tropical twist.
- Ginger: Swap with turmeric or cinnamon for a different flavor.

Dietary Needs and Allergies:
- Nut Allergy: Choose a non-nut milk alternative.
- Lactose Intolerance: Opt for lactose-free yogurt or non-dairy yogurt.
- Low-Carb: Reduce the amount of pineapple and use a lower-carb milk alternative.
- Diabetic-Friendly: Choose unsweetened coconut water and limit the fruit quantity.
- Allergic to Berries: Use sliced apples, peaches, or mango as a fruit alternative.

CHAPTER 2: GREEN ELIXIR

6. Kale Kiwi Kick

Ingredients:
- 1 cup kale, stems removed
- 2 ripe kiwis, peeled and sliced
- 1 stalk celery, chopped
- 1 cup green tea, cooled

Instructions:
1. Wash the kale and remove the stems.
2. Peel and slice the kiwis.
3. Chop the celery into smaller pieces.
4. Brew green tea and let it cool.
5. In a blender, combine the kale, kiwi slices, chopped celery, and cooled green tea.
6. Blend on high speed until the mixture is smooth and well combined.
7. Adjust the thickness by adding more green tea or water if necessary.
8. Pour the smoothie into a glass and serve.

Nutritional Information:
- Calories: Approximately 90 kcal
- Protein: 3g
- Fat: 1g
- Carbohydrates: 20g
- Fiber: 5g
- Sugar: 10g

Ingredient Substitutes:
- Kale: Substitute with spinach, Swiss chard, or collard greens.
- Kiwi: Use green apples or mango for a different fruity flavor.
- Celery: Replace with cucumber or zucchini for a milder taste.
- Green Tea: Swap with coconut water or almond milk for a different liquid base.

Dietary Needs and Allergies:
- Nut Allergy: Choose a non-nut milk alternative.
- Lactose Intolerance: Opt for lactose-free yogurt or non-dairy yogurt.
- Low-Carb: Reduce the amount of kiwi and choose low-carb liquid alternatives.
- Diabetic-Friendly: Choose unsweetened green tea and limit the fruit quantity.
- Allergic to Kiwi: Use strawberries, pineapple, or oranges as a fruit alternative.

7. Spinach Spirulina Splash

Ingredients:

- 1 cup fresh spinach leaves
- 1 teaspoon spirulina powder
- 1 cup pineapple, diced
- ½ cup cucumber, peeled and sliced

Instructions:

1. Wash the spinach leaves thoroughly.
2. Peel and dice the cucumber.
3. In a blender, combine the spinach, spirulina powder, pineapple, and cucumber.
4. Blend on high speed until the mixture is smooth and well combined.
5. Adjust the thickness by adding water or a liquid of your choice if needed.
6. Pour the smoothie into a glass and serve.

Nutritional Information:

- Calories: Approximately 120 kcal
- Protein: 5g
- Fat: 1g
- Carbohydrates: 25g
- Fiber: 8g
- Sugar: 15g

Ingredient Substitutes:
- Spinach: Swap with kale, Swiss chard, or collard greens.
- Spirulina: Replace with chlorella or wheatgrass for a different superfood boost.
- Pineapple: Use mango, peaches, or green apples for a tropical or slightly tart flavor.
- Cucumber: Swap with zucchini or celery for a milder taste.

Dietary Needs and Allergies:
- Nut Allergy: Choose a non-nut milk alternative.
- Lactose Intolerance: Opt for lactose-free yogurt or non-dairy yogurt.
- Low-Carb: Reduce the amount of pineapple and choose a low-carb liquid base.
- Diabetic-Friendly: Choose unsweetened liquid and limit the fruit quantity.
- Allergic to Tropical Fruits: Use berries, cherries, or stone fruits as pineapple alternatives.

8. Avocado Alchemy

Ingredients:

- 1 ripe avocado, peeled and pitted
- 1 cup arugula
- Juice of 1 lime
- 1 ½ cups coconut water

Instructions:

1. Peel and pit the ripe avocado.
2. In a blender, combine the avocado, arugula, lime juice, and coconut water.
3. Blend on high speed until the mixture is smooth and well combined.
4. Adjust the thickness by adding more coconut water if needed.
5. Pour the smoothie into a glass and serve.

Nutritional Information:

- Calories: Approximately 220 kcal
- Protein: 5g
- Fat: 15g
- Carbohydrates: 20g
- Fiber: 10g
- Sugar: 5g

Ingredient Substitutes:

- Avocado: Substitute with banana or Greek yogurt for a creamy texture.
- Arugula: Swap with spinach, kale, or Swiss chard.

- Lime: Replace with lemon for a citrusy twist.
- Coconut Water: Use almond milk, regular water, or green tea for a different liquid base.

Dietary Needs and Allergies:
- Nut Allergy: Choose a non-nut milk alternative.
- Lactose Intolerance: Opt for lactose-free yogurt or non-dairy yogurt.
- Low-Carb: Reduce the amount of avocado and choose a lower-carb liquid alternative.
- Diabetic-Friendly: Choose unsweetened liquid and limit the fruit quantity.
- Allergic to Citrus: Omit lime and use berries or pineapple for acidity.

9. Parsley Pineapple Potion

Ingredients:

- 1 cup pineapple, diced
- ½ cup fresh parsley leaves
- 1 green apple, cored and sliced
- 1 teaspoon fresh ginger, grated

Instructions:

1. Wash the parsley leaves and dice the pineapple.
2. Core and slice the green apple.
3. In a blender, combine the diced pineapple, fresh parsley leaves, sliced green apple, and grated ginger.
4. Blend on high speed until the mixture is smooth and well combined.
5. Adjust the thickness by adding water or a liquid of your choice if needed.
6. Pour the smoothie into a glass and serve.

Nutritional Information:

- Calories: Approximately 120 kcal
- Protein: 1g
- Fat: 0g
- Carbohydrates: 30g
- Fiber: 5g
- Sugar: 20g

Ingredient Substitutes:

- Pineapple: Swap with mango, peaches, or oranges for a tropical flavor.

- Parsley: Replace with cilantro or mint for a different herbaceous note.
- Green Apple: Use a red apple or pear for a sweeter taste.
- Ginger: Swap with turmeric or cinnamon for a different spice.

Dietary Needs and Allergies:
- Nut Allergy: Choose a non-nut milk alternative.
- Lactose Intolerance: Opt for lactose-free yogurt or non-dairy yogurt.
- Low-Carb: Reduce the amount of pineapple and choose a lower-carb liquid base.
- Diabetic-Friendly: Choose unsweetened liquid and limit the fruit quantity.

10. Cilantro Citrus Crush

Ingredients:

- 1 medium orange, peeled and segmented
- ½ cup fresh cilantro leaves
- ½ cup broccoli florets
- 1 ½ cups almond milk

Instructions:

1. Peel and segment the orange.
2. Wash the cilantro leaves and broccoli florets thoroughly.
3. In a blender, combine the orange segments, cilantro leaves, broccoli florets, and almond milk.
4. Blend on high speed until the mixture is smooth and well combined.
5. Adjust the thickness by adding more almond milk if needed.
6. Pour the smoothie into a glass and serve.

Nutritional Information:

- Calories: Approximately 120 kcal
- Protein: 3g
- Fat: 5g
- Carbohydrates: 18g
- Fiber: 6g
- Sugar: 10g

Ingredient Substitutes:

- Orange: Swap with grapefruit, mandarin, or pineapple for a different citrus flavor.

- Cilantro: Replace with mint or basil for a different herbaceous note.
- Broccoli: Use cauliflower or cucumber for a similar texture.
- Almond Milk: Swap with coconut milk, soy milk, or regular water for a different liquid base.

Dietary Needs and Allergies:
- Nut Allergy: Choose a non-nut milk alternative.
- Lactose Intolerance: Opt for lactose-free yogurt or non-dairy yogurt.
- Low-Carb: Reduce the amount of orange and choose a lower-carb liquid base.
- Diabetic-Friendly: Choose unsweetened liquid and limit the fruit quantity.
- Allergic to Citrus: Omit the orange and use berries or mango for acidity.

CHAPTER 3: TROPICAL TRANQUILITY

11. Papaya Paradise

Ingredients:

- 1 cup ripe papaya, peeled, seeded, and diced
- ½ teaspoon turmeric
- 1 cup mango, diced
- 1 ½ cups coconut water

Instructions:

1. Peel, seed, and dice the ripe papaya.
2. In a blender, combine the papaya, turmeric, mango, and coconut water.
3. Blend on high speed until the mixture is smooth and well combined.
4. Adjust the thickness by adding more coconut water if needed.
5. Pour the smoothie into a glass and serve.

Nutritional Information:

- Calories: Approximately 180 kcal
- Protein: 3g
- Fat: 1g
- Carbohydrates: 40g
- Fiber: 6g
- Sugar: 30g

Ingredient Substitutes:
- Papaya: Swap with peach, nectarine, or apricot for a similar texture.
- Turmeric: Replace with ginger or cinnamon for a different spice.
- Mango: Use pineapple, orange, or strawberries for a fruity alternative.
- Coconut Water: Swap with almond milk, pineapple juice, or regular water for a different liquid base.

Dietary Needs and Allergies:
- Nut Allergy: Choose a non-nut milk alternative.
- Lactose Intolerance: Opt for lactose-free yogurt or non-dairy yogurt.
- Low-Carb: Reduce the amount of papaya and choose a lower-carb liquid base.
- Diabetic-Friendly: Choose unsweetened liquid and limit the fruit quantity.

12. Passionfruit Pleasure

Ingredients:

- 2 passion fruits, scooped out
- 1 medium carrot, peeled and sliced
- 1 cup pineapple, diced
- ½ cup Greek yogurt

Instructions:

1. Scoop out the seeds from the passion fruits.
2. Peel and slice the carrot.
3. In a blender, combine the passion fruit seeds, sliced carrot, diced pineapple, and Greek yogurt.
4. Blend on high speed until the mixture is smooth and well combined.
5. Adjust the thickness by adding water or a liquid of your choice if needed.
6. Pour the smoothie into a glass and serve.

Nutritional Information:

- Calories: Approximately 150 kcal
- Protein: 6g
- Fat: 2g
- Carbohydrates: 30g
- Fiber: 5g
- Sugar: 20g

Ingredient Substitutes:

- Passionfruit: Swap with kiwi, mango, or pomegranate seeds for a burst of flavor.

- Carrot: Replace with cucumber, bell pepper, or sweet potato for a different vegetable base.
- Pineapple: Use orange, mango, or peaches for a tropical twist.
- Greek Yogurt: Swap with coconut milk yogurt or a non-dairy alternative for a different creamy texture.

Dietary Needs and Allergies:
- Nut Allergy: Choose a non-nut milk alternative.
- Lactose Intolerance: Opt for lactose-free yogurt or non-dairy yogurt.
- Low-Carb: Reduce the amount of pineapple and choose a lower-carb liquid base.
- Diabetic-Friendly: Choose unsweetened liquid and limit the fruit quantity.

13. Guava Glow

Ingredients:

- 1 cup guava, peeled and diced
- 1 cup spinach leaves
- 1 ripe banana
- 1 ½ cups coconut milk

Instructions:

1. Peel and dice the guava.
2. Wash the spinach leaves.
3. Peel the ripe banana.
4. In a blender, combine the guava, spinach leaves, banana, and coconut milk.
5. Blend on high speed until the mixture is smooth and well combined.
6. Adjust the thickness by adding more coconut milk if needed.
7. Pour the smoothie into a glass and serve.

Nutritional Information:

- Calories: Approximately 220 kcal
- Protein: 5g
- Fat: 10g
- Carbohydrates: 30g
- Fiber: 7g
- Sugar: 20g

Ingredient Substitutes:
- Guava: Swap with mango, pineapple, or strawberries for a different tropical flavor.
- Spinach: Replace with kale, Swiss chard, or collard greens.
- Banana: Use avocado or Greek yogurt for a creamy texture.
- Coconut Milk: Swap with almond milk, soy milk, or regular water for a different liquid base.

Dietary Needs and Allergies:
- Nut Allergy: Choose a non-nut milk alternative.
- Lactose Intolerance: Opt for lactose-free yogurt or non-dairy yogurt.
- Low-Carb: Reduce the amount of banana and choose a lower-carb liquid base.
- Diabetic-Friendly: Choose unsweetened liquid and limit the fruit quantity.

14. Dragon Fruit Dream

Ingredients:

- 1 cup dragon fruit, diced
- ½ cup lychee, peeled and pitted
- 1 handful mint leaves
- 1 ½ cups almond milk

Instructions:

1. Dice the dragon fruit.
2. Peel and pit the lychee.
3. In a blender, combine the diced dragon fruit, peeled lychee, mint leaves, and almond milk.
4. Blend on high speed until the mixture is smooth and well combined.
5. Adjust the thickness by adding more almond milk if needed.
6. Pour the smoothie into a glass and serve.

Nutritional Information:

- Calories: Approximately 150 kcal
- Protein: 3g
- Fat: 5g
- Carbohydrates: 25g
- Fiber: 7g
- Sugar: 15g

Ingredient Substitutes:

- Dragon Fruit: Swap with pitaya (pink dragon fruit) or mixed berries for a vibrant color.

- Lychee: Replace with pineapple, mango, or grapes for a sweet and juicy alternative.
- Mint Leaves: Use basil or cilantro for a different herbal note.
- Almond Milk: Swap with coconut milk, soy milk, or regular water for a different liquid base.

Dietary Needs and Allergies:
- Nut Allergy: Choose a non-nut milk alternative.
- Lactose Intolerance: Opt for lactose-free yogurt or non-dairy yogurt.
- Low-Carb: Reduce the amount of lychee and choose a lower-carb liquid base.
- Diabetic-Friendly: Choose unsweetened liquid and limit the fruit quantity.

15. Coconut Lime Oasis

Ingredients:

- 1 ½ cups coconut water
- Juice of 1 lime
- 1 cup pineapple, diced
- 1 cup kale, stems removed

Instructions:

1. In a blender, combine the coconut water, lime juice, diced pineapple, and kale.
2. Wash the kale thoroughly and remove the stems.
3. Blend on high speed until the mixture is smooth and well combined.
4. Adjust the thickness by adding more coconut water if needed.
5. Pour the smoothie into a glass and serve.

Nutritional Information:

- Calories: Approximately 90 kcal
- Protein: 3g
- Fat: 1g
- Carbohydrates: 25g
- Fiber: 5g
- Sugar: 15g

Ingredient Substitutes:

- Coconut Water: Swap with almond milk, regular water, or green tea for a different liquid base.
- Lime: Replace with lemon or grapefruit for a citrusy twist.

- Pineapple: Use mango, kiwi, or peaches for a tropical flavor.
- Kale: Swap with spinach, Swiss chard, or collard greens.

Dietary Needs and Allergies:
- Nut Allergy: Choose a non-nut milk alternative.
- Lactose Intolerance: Opt for lactose-free yogurt or non-dairy yogurt.
- Low-Carb: Reduce the amount of pineapple and choose a lower-carb liquid base.
- Diabetic-Friendly: Choose unsweetened liquid and limit the fruit quantity.

CHAPTER 4: SPICE SYMPHONY

16. Turmeric Tonic

Ingredients:
- 1 teaspoon turmeric
- 1 teaspoon fresh ginger, grated
- 1 cup mango, diced
- 1 medium carrot, peeled and sliced

Instructions:
1. Peel and dice the mango.
2. Peel and grate fresh ginger.
3. Peel and slice the carrot.
4. In a blender, combine the turmeric, grated ginger, diced mango, and sliced carrot.
5. Blend on high speed until the mixture is smooth and well combined.
6. Adjust the thickness by adding water or a liquid of your choice if needed.
7. Pour the smoothie into a glass and serve.

Nutritional Information:
- Calories: Approximately 120 kcal
- Protein: 2g
- Fat: 1g
- Carbohydrates: 30g
- Fiber: 6g
- Sugar: 18g

Ingredient Substitutes:
- Turmeric: Swap with cinnamon or cayenne pepper for a different spice.
- Ginger: Replace with ground ginger or turmeric for a different anti-inflammatory boost.
- Mango: Use pineapple, peaches, or apricots for a sweet and tropical flavor.
- Carrot: Swap with sweet potato or pumpkin for a similar texture.

Dietary Needs and Allergies:
- Nut Allergy: Choose a non-nut milk alternative.
- Lactose Intolerance: Opt for lactose-free yogurt or non-dairy yogurt.
- Low-Carb: Reduce the amount of mango and carrot and choose a lower-carb liquid base.
- Diabetic-Friendly: Choose unsweetened liquid and limit the fruit quantity.

17. Cinnamon Citrus Sip

Ingredients:
- 1 medium orange, peeled and segmented
- ½ teaspoon ground cinnamon
- 1 medium apple, cored and sliced
- 1 cup spinach leaves

Instructions:
1. Peel and segment the orange.
2. Wash the spinach leaves.
3. Core and slice the apple.
4. In a blender, combine the orange segments, ground cinnamon, sliced apple, and spinach leaves.
5. Blend on high speed until the mixture is smooth and well combined.
6. Adjust the thickness by adding more water or a liquid of your choice if needed.
7. Pour the smoothie into a glass and serve.

Nutritional Information:
- Calories: Approximately 120 kcal
- Protein: 2g
- Fat: 0g
- Carbohydrates: 30g
- Fiber: 7g
- Sugar: 20g

Ingredient Substitutes:
- Orange: Swap with grapefruit, mandarin, or pineapple for a different citrus flavor.
- Cinnamon: Replace with nutmeg or cardamom for a warm and aromatic spice.
- Apple: Use pear or berries for a different fruity taste.
- Spinach: Swap with kale, Swiss chard, or collard greens.

Dietary Needs and Allergies:
- Nut Allergy: Choose a non-nut milk alternative.
- Lactose Intolerance: Opt for lactose-free yogurt or non-dairy yogurt.
- Low-Carb: Reduce the amount of apple and choose a lower-carb liquid base.
- Diabetic-Friendly: Choose unsweetened liquid and limit the fruit quantity.

18. Cardamom Carrot Crush

Ingredients:

- 1 medium carrot, peeled and sliced
- ½ teaspoon ground cardamom
- 1 cup pineapple, diced
- ½ cup Greek yogurt

Instructions:

1. Peel and slice the carrot.
2. In a blender, combine the sliced carrot, ground cardamom, diced pineapple, and Greek yogurt.
3. Blend on high speed until the mixture is smooth and well combined.
4. Adjust the thickness by adding water or a liquid of your choice if needed.
5. Pour the smoothie into a glass and serve.

Nutritional Information:

- Calories: Approximately 120 kcal
- Protein: 5g
- Fat: 2g
- Carbohydrates: 25g
- Fiber: 5g
- Sugar: 15g

Ingredient Substitutes:

- Carrot: Swap with sweet potato or butternut squash for a similar texture.

- Cardamom: Replace with cinnamon or ginger for a different spice.
- Pineapple: Use mango, peaches, or apricots for a sweet and tropical flavor.
- Greek Yogurt: Choose coconut milk yogurt or a non-dairy alternative for a different creamy texture.

Dietary Needs and Allergies:
- Nut Allergy: Choose a non-nut milk alternative.
- Lactose Intolerance: Opt for lactose-free yogurt or non-dairy yogurt.
- Low-Carb: Reduce the amount of pineapple and choose a lower-carb liquid base.
- Diabetic-Friendly: Choose unsweetened liquid and limit the fruit quantity.

19. Cayenne Mango Mojo

Ingredients:

- 1 cup mango, diced
- ⅛ teaspoon cayenne pepper
- ½ cup cucumber, peeled and sliced
- 1 ½ cups coconut water

Instructions:

1. Peel and dice the mango.
2. Peel and slice the cucumber.
3. In a blender, combine the diced mango, cayenne pepper, sliced cucumber, and coconut water.
4. Blend on high speed until the mixture is smooth and well combined.
5. Adjust the thickness by adding more coconut water if needed.
6. Pour the smoothie into a glass and serve.

Nutritional Information:

- Calories: Approximately 100 kcal
- Protein: 2g
- Fat: 0g
- Carbohydrates: 25g
- Fiber: 5g
- Sugar: 18g

Ingredient Substitutes:

- Mango: Swap with pineapple, peaches, or apricots for a sweet and tropical flavor.

- Cayenne Pepper: Replace with chili powder or a pinch of black pepper for a different level of heat.
- Cucumber: Use zucchini or celery for a milder taste.
- Coconut Water: Swap with almond milk, regular water, or green tea for a different liquid base.

Dietary Needs and Allergies:
- Nut Allergy: Choose a non-nut milk alternative.
- Lactose Intolerance: Opt for lactose-free yogurt or non-dairy yogurt.
- Low-Carb: Reduce the amount of mango and choose a lower-carb liquid base.
- Diabetic-Friendly: Choose unsweetened liquid and limit the fruit quantity.

20. Rosemary Berry Blast

Ingredients:

- 1 cup blueberries
- 1 teaspoon fresh rosemary leaves
- 1 ripe banana
- 1 ½ cups almond milk

Instructions:

1. Wash the blueberries and remove any stems.
2. Peel the ripe banana.
3. In a blender, combine the blueberries, fresh rosemary leaves, ripe banana, and almond milk.
4. Blend on high speed until the mixture is smooth and well combined.
5. Adjust the thickness by adding more almond milk if needed.
6. Pour the smoothie into a glass and serve.

Nutritional Information:

- Calories: Approximately 180 kcal
- Protein: 3g
- Fat: 3g
- Carbohydrates: 40g
- Fiber: 8g
- Sugar: 22g

Ingredient Substitutes:

- Blueberries: Swap with raspberries, blackberries, or strawberries.

- Rosemary: Replace with thyme or mint for a different herbal note.
- Banana: Use avocado or Greek yogurt for a creamy texture.
- Almond Milk: Swap with coconut milk, soy milk, or regular water for a different liquid base.

Dietary Needs and Allergies:
- Nut Allergy: Choose a non-nut milk alternative.
- Lactose Intolerance: Opt for lactose-free yogurt or non-dairy yogurt.
- Low-Carb: Reduce the amount of banana and choose a lower-carb liquid base.
- Diabetic-Friendly: Choose unsweetened liquid and limit the fruit quantity.

CHAPTER 5: CITRUS SYMPHONY
21. Lemon Lavender Lift
Ingredients:
- 1 medium lemon, peeled and segmented
- 1 teaspoon dried lavender flowers
- 1 cup pineapple, diced
- 1 cup kale, stems removed

Instructions:
1. Peel and segment the lemon.
2. In a blender, combine the lemon segments, dried lavender flowers, diced pineapple, and kale.
3. Wash the kale thoroughly and remove the stems.
4. Blend on high speed until the mixture is smooth and well combined.
5. Adjust the thickness by adding more coconut water or a liquid of your choice if needed.
6. Pour the smoothie into a glass and serve.

Nutritional Information:
- Calories: Approximately 100 kcal
- Protein: 3g
- Fat: 1g
- Carbohydrates: 25g
- Fiber: 6g
- Sugar: 15g

Ingredient Substitutes:
- Lemon: Swap with lime or grapefruit for a different citrus flavor.
- Lavender: Replace with mint or chamomile for a different herbal note.
- Pineapple: Use mango, peaches, or apricots for a sweet and tropical flavor.
- Kale: Swap with spinach, Swiss chard, or collard greens.

Dietary Needs and Allergies:
- Nut Allergy: Choose a non-nut milk alternative.
- Lactose Intolerance: Opt for lactose-free yogurt or non-dairy yogurt.
- Low-Carb: Reduce the amount of pineapple and choose a lower-carb liquid base.
- Diabetic-Friendly: Choose unsweetened liquid and limit the fruit quantity.

22. Orange Ginger Zest

Ingredients:

- 1 medium orange, peeled and segmented
- 1 teaspoon fresh ginger, grated
- 1 medium carrot, peeled and sliced
- 1 ½ cups coconut water

Instructions:

1. Peel and segment the orange.
2. Peel and grate fresh ginger.
3. Peel and slice the carrot.
4. In a blender, combine the orange segments, grated ginger, sliced carrot, and coconut water.
5. Blend on high speed until the mixture is smooth and well mixed.
6. Adjust the thickness by adding more coconut water if needed.
7. Pour the smoothie into a glass and serve.

Nutritional Information:

- Calories: Approximately 120 kcal
- Protein: 2g
- Fat: 0g
- Carbohydrates: 30g
- Fiber: 5g
- Sugar: 20g

Ingredient Substitutes:
- Orange: Swap with grapefruit, mandarin, or pineapple for a different citrus flavor.
- Ginger: Replace with turmeric or cayenne pepper for a different spice.
- Carrot: Use sweet potato or pumpkin for a similar texture.
- Coconut Water: Swap with almond milk, regular water, or green tea for a different liquid base.

Dietary Needs and Allergies:
- Nut Allergy: Choose a non-nut milk alternative.
- Lactose Intolerance: Opt for lactose-free yogurt or non-dairy yogurt.
- Low-Carb: Reduce the amount of orange and choose a lower-carb liquid base.
- Diabetic-Friendly: Choose unsweetened liquid and limit the fruit quantity.

23. Grapefruit Green Goddess

Ingredients:

- 1 medium grapefruit, peeled and segmented
- 1 cup spinach leaves
- 1 handful mint leaves
- 1 cup cucumber, peeled and sliced

Instructions:

1. Peel and segment the grapefruit.
2. Wash the spinach leaves, mint leaves, and cucumber.
3. In a blender, combine the grapefruit segments, spinach leaves, mint leaves, and sliced cucumber.
4. Blend on high speed until the mixture is smooth and well mixed.
5. Adjust the thickness by adding more coconut water or a liquid of your choice if needed.
6. Pour the smoothie into a glass and serve.

Nutritional Information:

- Calories: Approximately 90 kcal
- Protein: 2g
- Fat: 1g
- Carbohydrates: 20g
- Fiber: 5g
- Sugar: 10g

Ingredient Substitutes:

- Grapefruit: Swap with orange or pineapple for a different citrus flavor.

- Spinach: Replace with kale, Swiss chard, or collard greens.
- Mint Leaves: Use cilantro or basil for a different herbal note.
- Cucumber: Swap with celery or zucchini for a milder taste.

Dietary Needs and Allergies:
- Nut Allergy: Choose a non-nut milk alternative.
- Lactose Intolerance: Opt for lactose-free yogurt or non-dairy yogurt.
- Low-Carb: Reduce the amount of grapefruit and choose a lower-carb liquid base.
- Diabetic-Friendly: Choose unsweetened liquid and limit the fruit quantity.

24. Citrus Basil Bliss

Ingredients:
- 1 medium lime, peeled and segmented
- 1 handful fresh basil leaves
- 1 cup pineapple, diced
- 1 ½ cups coconut milk

Instructions:
1. Peel and segment the lime.
2. Wash the fresh basil leaves.
3. In a blender, combine the lime segments, fresh basil leaves, diced pineapple, and coconut milk.
4. Blend on high speed until the mixture is smooth and well combined.
5. Adjust the thickness by adding more coconut milk if needed.
6. Pour the smoothie into a glass and serve.

Nutritional Information:
- Calories: Approximately 160 kcal
- Protein: 2g
- Fat: 5g
- Carbohydrates: 30g
- Fiber: 6g
- Sugar: 20g

Ingredient Substitutes:
- Lime: Swap with lemon or orange for a different citrus flavor.

- Basil: Replace with mint or cilantro for a different herbal note.
- Pineapple: Use mango, peaches, or apricots for a sweet and tropical flavor.
- Coconut Milk: Swap with almond milk, soy milk, or regular water for a different liquid base.

Dietary Needs and Allergies:
- Nut Allergy: Choose a non-nut milk alternative.
- Lactose Intolerance: Opt for lactose-free yogurt or non-dairy yogurt.
- Low-Carb: Reduce the amount of pineapple and choose a lower-carb liquid base.
- Diabetic-Friendly: Choose unsweetened liquid and limit the fruit quantity.

25. Tangerine Turmeric Twist

Ingredients:

- 2 medium tangerines, peeled and segmented
- 1 teaspoon turmeric
- 1 cup mango, diced
- 1 ½ cups almond milk

Instructions:

1. Peel and segment the tangerines.
2. In a blender, combine the tangerine segments, turmeric, diced mango, and almond milk.
3. Blend on high speed until the mixture is smooth and well combined.
4. Adjust the thickness by adding more almond milk if needed.
5. Pour the smoothie into a glass and serve.

Nutritional Information:

- Calories: Approximately 140 kcal
- Protein: 3g
- Fat: 3g
- Carbohydrates: 30g
- Fiber: 6g
- Sugar: 20g

Ingredient Substitutes:

- Tangerine: Swap with orange or mandarin for a different citrus flavor.

- Turmeric: Replace with ginger or cinnamon for a different spice.
- Mango: Use pineapple, peaches, or apricots for a sweet and tropical flavor.
- Almond Milk: Swap with coconut milk, soy milk, or regular water for a different liquid base.

Dietary Needs and Allergies:
- Nut Allergy: Choose a non-nut milk alternative.
- Lactose Intolerance: Opt for lactose-free yogurt or non-dairy yogurt.
- Low-Carb: Reduce the amount of mango and choose a lower-carb liquid base.
- Diabetic-Friendly: Choose unsweetened liquid and limit the fruit quantity.

CHAPTER 6: NUTTY NIRVANA

26. Almond Joy Delight

Ingredients:

- 2 tablespoons almond butter
- 1 ½ cups coconut water
- 1 ripe banana
- 1 cup spinach leaves

Instructions:

1. Peel the ripe banana.
2. In a blender, combine the almond butter, coconut water, peeled banana, and spinach leaves.
3. Wash the spinach leaves thoroughly.
4. Blend on high speed until the mixture is smooth and well combined.
5. Adjust the thickness by adding more coconut water if needed.
6. Pour the smoothie into a glass and serve.

Nutritional Information:

- Calories: Approximately 220 kcal
- Protein: 5g
- Fat: 15g
- Carbohydrates: 20g
- Fiber: 5g
- Sugar: 10g

Ingredient Substitutes:
- Almond Butter: Swap with peanut butter, sunflower seed butter, or tahini.
- Coconut Water: Replace with almond milk, regular water, or green tea for a different liquid base.
- Banana: Use mango or avocado for a creamy texture.
- Spinach: Swap with kale, Swiss chard, or collard greens.

Dietary Needs and Allergies:
- Nut Allergy: Choose a non-nut butter alternative.
- Lactose Intolerance: Opt for lactose-free yogurt or non-dairy yogurt.
- Low-Carb: Reduce the amount of banana and choose a lower-carb liquid base.
- Diabetic-Friendly: Choose unsweetened liquid and limit the fruit quantity.

27. Walnut Wonder

Ingredients:
- ¼ cup walnuts
- 1 cup blueberries
- 1 cup kale, stems removed
- ½ cup Greek yogurt

Instructions:
1. Wash the blueberries and remove any stems.
2. In a blender, combine the walnuts, blueberries, washed kale, and Greek yogurt.
3. Remove the stems from the kale.
4. Blend on high speed until the mixture is smooth and well combined.
5. Adjust the thickness by adding more water or a liquid of your choice if needed.
6. Pour the smoothie into a glass and serve.

Nutritional Information:
- Calories: Approximately 250 kcal
- Protein: 10g
- Fat: 15g
- Carbohydrates: 25g
- Fiber: 6g
- Sugar: 15g

Ingredient Substitutes:
- Walnuts: Swap with almonds, pecans, or sunflower seeds.
- Blueberries: Use raspberries, blackberries, or strawberries.

- Kale: Swap with spinach, Swiss chard, or collard greens.
- Greek Yogurt: Choose coconut milk yogurt or a non-dairy alternative for a different creamy texture.

Dietary Needs and Allergies:
- Nut Allergy: Choose a nut-free seed or butter alternative.
- Lactose Intolerance: Opt for lactose-free yogurt or non-dairy yogurt.
- Low-Carb: Reduce the amount of blueberries and choose a lower-carb liquid base.
- Diabetic-Friendly: Choose unsweetened liquid and limit the fruit quantity.

28. Cashew Cherry Charm

Ingredients:

- ¼ cup cashews
- 1 cup cherries, pitted
- ½ small beetroot, peeled and diced
- 1 ½ cups coconut milk

Instructions:

1. Pit the cherries.
2. Peel and dice the beetroot.
3. In a blender, combine the cashews, pitted cherries, diced beetroot, and coconut milk.
4. Blend on high speed until the mixture is smooth and well combined.
5. Adjust the thickness by adding more coconut milk if needed.
6. Pour the smoothie into a glass and serve.

Nutritional Information:

- Calories: Approximately 220 kcal
- Protein: 5g
- Fat: 10g
- Carbohydrates: 30g
- Fiber: 7g
- Sugar: 15g

Ingredient Substitutes:

- Cashews: Swap with almonds, walnuts, or sunflower seeds.
- Cherries: Use raspberries, blackberries, or strawberries.

- Beetroot: Replace with carrot for a similar color and texture.
- Coconut Milk: Swap with almond milk, soy milk, or regular water for a different liquid base.

Dietary Needs and Allergies:
- Nut Allergy: Choose a nut-free seed alternative.
- Lactose Intolerance: Opt for lactose-free yogurt or non-dairy yogurt.
- Low-Carb: Reduce the amount of cherries and choose a lower-carb liquid base.
- Diabetic-Friendly: Choose unsweetened liquid and limit the fruit quantity.

29. Pecan Pumpkin Pleasure

Ingredients:

- ¼ cup pecans
- ½ cup pumpkin puree
- ½ teaspoon cinnamon
- ½ cup Greek yogurt

Instructions:

1. In a blender, combine the pecans, pumpkin puree, cinnamon, and Greek yogurt.
2. Blend on high speed until the mixture is smooth and well combined.
3. Adjust the thickness by adding more water or a liquid of your choice if needed.
4. Pour the smoothie into a glass and serve.

Nutritional Information:

- Calories: Approximately 220 kcal
- Protein: 10g
- Fat: 15g
- Carbohydrates: 20g
- Fiber: 6g
- Sugar: 10g

Ingredient Substitutes:

- Pecans: Swap with walnuts, almonds, or hazelnuts.
- Pumpkin Puree: Use sweet potato puree or butternut squash for a similar texture.

- Cinnamon: Replace with nutmeg or pumpkin spice for a different spice.
- Greek Yogurt: Choose coconut milk yogurt or a non-dairy alternative for a different creamy texture.

Dietary Needs and Allergies:
- Nut Allergy: Choose a nut-free seed alternative.
- Lactose Intolerance: Opt for lactose-free yogurt or non-dairy yogurt.
- Low-Carb: Reduce the amount of pumpkin puree and choose a lower-carb liquid base.
- Diabetic-Friendly: Choose unsweetened liquid and limit the fruit quantity.

30. Hazelnut Hibiscus Hug

Ingredients:

- ¼ cup hazelnuts
- 1 cup hibiscus tea, cooled
- 1 cup raspberries
- 1 cup spinach leaves

Instructions:

1. Brew hibiscus tea and let it cool to room temperature.
2. In a blender, combine the hazelnuts, cooled hibiscus tea, raspberries, and spinach leaves.
3. Wash the spinach leaves thoroughly.
4. Blend on high speed until the mixture is smooth and well combined.
5. Adjust the thickness by adding more hibiscus tea if needed.
6. Pour the smoothie into a glass and serve.

Nutritional Information:

- Calories: Approximately 150 kcal
- Protein: 4g
- Fat: 9g
- Carbohydrates: 18g
- Fiber: 7g
- Sugar: 7g

Ingredient Substitutes:

- Hazelnuts: Swap with almonds, walnuts, or sunflower seeds.

- Hibiscus Tea: Replace with green tea or a herbal tea of your choice for a different flavor.
- Raspberries: Use blackberries, strawberries, or blueberries.
- Spinach: Swap with kale, Swiss chard, or collard greens.

Dietary Needs and Allergies:
- Nut Allergy: Choose a nut-free seed alternative.
- Low-Carb: Reduce the amount of raspberries and choose a lower-carb liquid base.
- Diabetic-Friendly: Choose unsweetened tea and limit the fruit quantity.

CHAPTER 7: HERBAL INFUSION

31. Peppermint Pineapple Paradise

Ingredients:

- 1 teaspoon fresh peppermint leaves
- 1 cup pineapple, diced
- 1 ripe banana
- 1 ½ cups coconut water

Instructions:

1. Wash the fresh peppermint leaves.
2. Peel the ripe banana.
3. In a blender, combine the fresh peppermint leaves, diced pineapple, peeled banana, and coconut water.
4. Blend on high speed until the mixture is smooth and well combined.
5. Adjust the thickness by adding more coconut water if needed.
6. Pour the smoothie into a glass and serve.

Nutritional Information:

- Calories: Approximately 150 kcal
- Protein: 2g
- Fat: 0g
- Carbohydrates: 35g
- Fiber: 5g
- Sugar: 20g

Ingredient Substitutes:
- Peppermint: Swap with fresh basil or cilantro for a different herbal note.
- Pineapple: Use mango, peaches, or apricots for a sweet and tropical flavor.
- Banana: Use avocado for a creamy texture.
- Coconut Water: Swap with almond milk, soy milk, or regular water for a different liquid base.

Dietary Needs and Allergies:
- Nut Allergy: Choose a nut-free seed alternative.
- Lactose Intolerance: Opt for lactose-free yogurt or non-dairy yogurt.
- Low-Carb: Reduce the amount of banana and choose a lower-carb liquid base.
- Diabetic-Friendly: Choose unsweetened liquid and limit the fruit quantity.

32. Chamomile Citrus Soothe

Ingredients:

- 1 cup chamomile tea, cooled
- 1 medium orange, peeled and segmented
- 1 cup mango, diced
- 1 cup spinach leaves

Instructions:

1. Brew chamomile tea and let it cool to room temperature.
2. Peel and segment the orange.
3. In a blender, combine the cooled chamomile tea, orange segments, diced mango, and spinach leaves.
4. Wash the spinach leaves thoroughly.
5. Blend on high speed until the mixture is smooth and well combined.
6. Adjust the thickness by adding more chamomile tea if needed.
7. Pour the smoothie into a glass and serve.

Nutritional Information:

- Calories: Approximately 120 kcal
- Protein: 2g
- Fat: 1g
- Carbohydrates: 28g
- Fiber: 5g
- Sugar: 20g

Ingredient Substitutes:
- Chamomile Tea: Replace with green tea or a herbal tea of your choice for a different flavor.
- Orange: Swap with grapefruit or mandarin for a different citrus flavor.
- Mango: Use pineapple, peaches, or apricots for a sweet and tropical flavor.
- Spinach: Swap with kale, Swiss chard, or collard greens.

Dietary Needs and Allergies:
- Nut Allergy: Choose a nut-free seed alternative.
- Lactose Intolerance: Opt for lactose-free yogurt or non-dairy yogurt.
- Low-Carb: Reduce the amount of mango and choose a lower-carb liquid base.
- Diabetic-Friendly: Choose unsweetened liquid and limit the fruit quantity.

33. Lemongrass Lime Lullaby

Ingredients:

- 1 stalk lemongrass, chopped
- 1 medium lime, peeled and segmented
- 1 cup pineapple, diced
- 1 cup cucumber, peeled and sliced

Instructions:

1. Peel and segment the lime.
2. Peel and dice the cucumber.
3. In a blender, combine the chopped lemongrass, lime segments, diced pineapple, and sliced cucumber.
4. Blend on high speed until the mixture is smooth and well combined.
5. Adjust the thickness by adding more coconut water or a liquid of your choice if needed.
6. Pour the smoothie into a glass and serve.

Nutritional Information:

- Calories: Approximately 90 kcal
- Protein: 2g
- Fat: 1g
- Carbohydrates: 22g
- Fiber: 5g
- Sugar: 12g

Ingredient Substitutes:

- Lemongrass: Swap with fresh mint or cilantro for a different herbal note.

- Lime: Replace with lemon or grapefruit for a different citrus flavor.
- Pineapple: Use mango, peaches, or apricots for a sweet and tropical flavor.
- Cucumber: Swap with celery or zucchini for a milder taste.

Dietary Needs and Allergies:
- Nut Allergy: Choose a nut-free seed alternative.
- Low-Carb: Reduce the amount of pineapple and choose a lower-carb liquid base.
- Diabetic-Friendly: Choose unsweetened liquid and limit the fruit quantity.

34. Basil Berry Breeze

Ingredients:

- 1 cup fresh basil leaves
- 1 cup blueberries
- 1 cup strawberries, hulled
- 1 ½ cups coconut milk

Instructions:

1. Wash the fresh basil leaves.
2. Hull the strawberries.
3. In a blender, combine the fresh basil leaves, blueberries, hulled strawberries, and coconut milk.
4. Blend on high speed until the mixture is smooth and well combined.
5. Adjust the thickness by adding more coconut milk if needed.
6. Pour the smoothie into a glass and serve.

Nutritional Information:

- Calories: Approximately 160 kcal
- Protein: 2g
- Fat: 5g
- Carbohydrates: 30g
- Fiber: 8g
- Sugar: 15g

Ingredient Substitutes:

- Basil: Swap with mint or cilantro for a different herbal note.
- Blueberries: Use raspberries, blackberries, or strawberries.

- Strawberries: Replace with mango or peaches for a sweet and tropical flavor.
- Coconut Milk: Swap with almond milk, soy milk, or regular water for a different liquid base.

Dietary Needs and Allergies:
- Nut Allergy: Choose a nut-free seed alternative.
- Lactose Intolerance: Opt for lactose-free yogurt or non-dairy yogurt.
- Low-Carb: Reduce the amount of strawberries and choose a lower-carb liquid base.
- Diabetic-Friendly: Choose unsweetened liquid and limit the fruit quantity.

35. Rosehip Raspberry Relaxation

Ingredients:

- 1 cup rosehip tea, cooled
- 1 cup raspberries
- 1 ripe banana
- 1 ½ cups almond milk

Instructions:

1. Brew rosehip tea and let it cool to room temperature.
2. In a blender, combine the cooled rosehip tea, raspberries, peeled banana, and almond milk.
3. Peel the ripe banana.
4. Blend on high speed until the mixture is smooth and well combined.
5. Adjust the thickness by adding more almond milk if needed.
6. Pour the smoothie into a glass and serve.

Nutritional Information:

- Calories: Approximately 120 kcal
- Protein: 3g
- Fat: 3g
- Carbohydrates: 25g
- Fiber: 8g
- Sugar: 12g

Ingredient Substitutes:

- Rosehip Tea: Replace with hibiscus tea or green tea for a different flavor.

- Raspberries: Use blackberries, strawberries, or blueberries.
- Banana: Swap with mango or avocado for a creamy texture.
- Almond Milk: Swap with coconut milk, soy milk, or regular water for a different liquid base.

Dietary Needs and Allergies:
- Nut Allergy: Choose a nut-free seed alternative.
- Lactose Intolerance: Opt for lactose-free yogurt or non-dairy yogurt.
- Low-Carb: Reduce the amount of banana and choose a lower-carb liquid base.
- Diabetic-Friendly: Choose unsweetened tea and limit the fruit quantity.

CHAPTER 8: FLORAL FUSION

36. Hibiscus Honey Harmony

Ingredients:
- 1 tablespoon dried hibiscus petals
- 1 tablespoon honey
- 1 cup mango, diced
- 1 cup spinach leaves

Instructions:
1. Brew hibiscus tea by steeping dried hibiscus petals in hot water for 5 minutes and let it cool.
2. In a blender, combine the cooled hibiscus tea (without petals), honey, diced mango, and spinach leaves.
3. Wash the spinach leaves thoroughly.
4. Blend on high speed until the mixture is smooth and well combined.
5. Adjust the thickness by adding more hibiscus tea or a liquid of your choice if needed.
6. Pour the smoothie into a glass and serve.

Nutritional Information:
- Calories: Approximately 120 kcal
- Protein: 2g
- Fat: 0g
- Carbohydrates: 30g
- Fiber: 5g
- Sugar: 20g

Ingredient Substitutes:
- Hibiscus Petals: Replace with hibiscus tea bags for convenience or use another herbal tea.
- Honey: Swap with maple syrup or agave nectar for a different natural sweetener.
- Mango: Use peaches, apricots, or pineapple for a sweet and tropical flavor.
- Spinach: Swap with kale, Swiss chard, or collard greens.

Dietary Needs and Allergies:
- Nut Allergy: Choose a nut-free seed alternative.
- Low-Carb: Reduce the amount of mango and choose a lower-carb liquid base.
- Diabetic-Friendly: Choose unsweetened tea and limit the fruit quantity.

37. Lavender Lemonade Lift

Ingredients:

- 1 teaspoon dried lavender flowers
- 1 medium lemon, peeled and segmented
- 1 cup pineapple, diced
- 1 cup kale, stems removed

Instructions:

1. Peel and segment the lemon.
2. In a blender, combine the dried lavender flowers, lemon segments, diced pineapple, and kale.
3. Wash the kale thoroughly and remove the stems.
4. Blend on high speed until the mixture is smooth and well combined.
5. Adjust the thickness by adding more coconut water or a liquid of your choice if needed.
6. Pour the smoothie into a glass and serve.

Nutritional Information:

- Calories: Approximately 120 kcal
- Protein: 3g
- Fat: 1g
- Carbohydrates: 30g
- Fiber: 6g
- Sugar: 15g

Ingredient Substitutes:

- Lavender: Replace with mint or chamomile for a different herbal note.

- Lemon: Swap with lime or grapefruit for a different citrus flavor.
- Pineapple: Use mango, peaches, or apricots for a sweet and tropical flavor.
- Kale: Swap with spinach, Swiss chard, or collard greens.

Dietary Needs and Allergies:
- Nut Allergy: Choose a nut-free seed alternative.
- Low-Carb: Reduce the amount of pineapple and choose a lower-carb liquid base.
- Diabetic-Friendly: Choose unsweetened liquid and limit the fruit quantity.

38. Rose Petal Radiance

Ingredients:
- 1 tablespoon rose petals (culinary grade)
- 1 cup raspberries
- 1 ripe banana
- 1 ½ cups coconut milk

Instructions:
1. In a blender, combine the rose petals, raspberries, peeled banana, and coconut milk.
2. Peel the ripe banana.
3. Blend on high speed until the mixture is smooth and well combined.
4. Adjust the thickness by adding more coconut milk if needed.
5. Pour the smoothie into a glass and serve immediately.

Nutritional Information:
- Calories: Approximately 140 kcal
- Protein: 2g
- Fat: 5g
- Carbohydrates: 25g
- Fiber: 8g
- Sugar: 12g

Ingredient Substitutes:
- Rose Petals: Replace with hibiscus petals or another edible flower for a different floral note.
- Raspberries: Use blackberries, strawberries, or blueberries.

- Banana: Swap with mango or avocado for a creamy texture.
- Coconut Milk: Swap with almond milk, soy milk, or regular water for a different liquid base.

Dietary Needs and Allergies:
- Nut Allergy: Choose a nut-free seed alternative.
- Low-Carb: Reduce the amount of banana and choose a lower-carb liquid base.
- Diabetic-Friendly: Choose unsweetened liquid and limit the fruit quantity.

39. Chamomile Vanilla Velvet

Ingredients:
- 1 cup chamomile tea, cooled
- ½ teaspoon vanilla extract
- 1 cup peach, diced
- 1 ½ cups almond milk

Instructions:
1. Brew chamomile tea and let it cool to room temperature.
2. In a blender, combine the cooled chamomile tea, vanilla extract, diced peach, and almond milk.
3. Peel and dice the peach.
4. Blend on high speed until the mixture is smooth and well combined.
5. Adjust the thickness by adding more chamomile tea if needed.
6. Pour the smoothie into a glass and serve.

Nutritional Information:
- Calories: Approximately 120 kcal
- Protein: 3g
- Fat: 2g
- Carbohydrates: 25g
- Fiber: 6g
- Sugar: 18g

Ingredient Substitutes:
- Chamomile Tea: Replace with green tea or a herbal tea of your choice for a different flavor.

- Vanilla Extract: Use ground vanilla bean or skip for a milder vanilla flavor.
- Peach: Swap with apricots, mango, or nectarines for a sweet and fruity flavor.
- Almond Milk: Swap with coconut milk, soy milk, or regular water for a different liquid base.

Dietary Needs and Allergies:
- Nut Allergy: Choose a nut-free seed alternative.
- Low-Carb: Reduce the amount of peach and choose a lower-carb liquid base.
- Diabetic-Friendly: Choose unsweetened tea and limit the fruit quantity.

40. Jasmine Ginger Jazz

Ingredients:

- 1 cup jasmine tea, cooled
- 1 teaspoon fresh ginger, grated
- 1 cup blueberries
- 1 ½ cups coconut water

Instructions:

1. Brew jasmine tea and let it cool to room temperature.
2. Peel and grate the fresh ginger.
3. In a blender, combine the cooled jasmine tea, grated ginger, blueberries, and coconut water.
4. Wash the blueberries thoroughly.
5. Blend on high speed until the mixture is smooth and well combined.
6. Adjust the thickness by adding more coconut water if needed.
7. Pour the smoothie into a glass and serve.

Nutritional Information:

- Calories: Approximately 100 kcal
- Protein: 2g
- Fat: 0g
- Carbohydrates: 25g
- Fiber: 5g
- Sugar: 15g

Ingredient Substitutes:
- Jasmine Tea: Replace with green tea or a herbal tea of your choice for a different flavor.
- Ginger: Swap with ground ginger or turmeric for a different spice.
- Blueberries: Use raspberries, blackberries, or strawberries.
- Coconut Water: Swap with almond milk, soy milk, or regular water for a different liquid base.

Dietary Needs and Allergies:
- Nut Allergy: Choose a nut-free seed alternative.
- Low-Carb: Reduce the amount of blueberries and choose a lower-carb liquid base.
- Diabetic-Friendly: Choose unsweetened tea and limit the fruit quantity.

Enjoy experimenting with these flavorful and nutritious anti-inflammatory smoothies!

CONCLUSION
Thrive On, Wellness Seekers

As we bid farewell to "*Anti-Inflammatory Smoothie*" by Aveline Winter, let's not view it as an ending but rather a commencement – a commencement of a transformative wellness journey. Aveline's meticulous crafting of these recipes isn't just a culinary adventure; it's an invitation to embrace well-being with every sip.

You've navigated through the vivid Blueberry Burst, the calming Rose Petal Radiance, and an array of other tantalizing concoctions, each designed to alleviate discomfort and elevate your vitality. The journey doesn't conclude with the final page; it extends into your kitchen, into each blending session, and ultimately, into the vibrant life you're crafting.

These recipes are more than a blend of ingredients; they're a commitment to your health. Every detailed ingredient list, each nutritional insight, and the thoughtful consideration for substitutes demonstrate Aveline's dedication to your well-being. It's a guide, not just to delicious smoothies, but to a lifestyle that cherishes your health.

As you close this book, don't perceive it as a conclusion. See it as a call to action – a call to keep pushing, to keep experimenting, and to keep prioritizing your health. The power to thrive is in your hands, and the journey ahead is yours to shape.

So, keep pushing. Keep blending. Keep sipping your way to a healthier, happier you. This isn't the end; it's a new beginning. Your wellness journey is ongoing, and the pages you write with every smoothie are a testament to your commitment to self-care.

Thriving isn't a destination; it's a continuous pursuit. Keep pushing, keep savoring, and keep thriving. Your well-being is worth every vibrant sip. Here's to a future filled with health, joy, and the zest of life.

Keep pushing – I'm rooting for you.

A HEARTFELT THANK YOU!

Thank you for your support on this culinary journey! If you enjoyed this book, please consider creating a video review or, if that's not feasible, leaving a written review. You can include a picture of the book or a page that caught your interest.

STEPS ON HOW TO LEAVE A REVIEW FOR THIS BOOK

1. Scan the QR code with your phone camera, a link will pop up on your screen, simply click on it to visit my author page.

2. Scroll down and locate the book titled "ANTI-INFLAMMATORY SMOOTHIE" by Aveline Winter.

3. Once you find the book, click on its title to navigate to the book's sales page.

4. Scroll down on the sales page, and right after the "About the Author" section, you'll find the "Customer Reviews" section.

5. In the "Customer Reviews" section, you'll see an option to leave a review. Begin by rating the book with stars, indicating your overall satisfaction with it.

6. After rating, a text box or prompt will appear for you to leave a written review. Share your thoughts, experiences, and any feedback you have about the book.

7. Once you've written your review, double-check to ensure everything looks good, and then submit your review.

Your feedback is invaluable and greatly appreciated!
Thank you for taking the time to share your thoughts on
"ANTI-INFLAMMATORY SMOOTHIE."